BEING A MAN

By

Ben Jackson & Sam Lawrence

Disclaimer

DiAll attempts have been made to verify the information contained in this book but the author and publisher do not bear any responsibility for errors or omissions. Any perceived negative connotation of any individual, group, or company is purely unintentional. Furthermore, this book is intended as entertainment only and as such, any and all responsibility for actions taken upon reading this book lies with the reader alone and not with the author or publisher. This book is not intended as medical, legal, or business advice and the reader alone holds sole responsibility for any consequences of any actions taken after reading this book. Additionally, it is the reader's responsibility alone and not the author's or publisher's to ensure that all applicable laws and regulations for business practice are adhered to.

Published by Indie Publishing Group

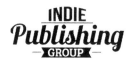

TABLE OF CONTENTS

INTRODUCTION

WELCOME ONE AND all to the Ben and Sam show. Well that's what it feels like at times believe me. We both met over two years ago and we are currently in a long distance relationship, she lives in Canada and I'm from Australia. So, if you notice any weird mannerisms in our speech that's where they come from. We set out to write this book together with input from both of us in all chapters. Sometimes you will see comments from Sam, sometimes from Ben. The intent of this book is to provide as many general tips/hacks for men without getting seriously bogged down into one particular subject. We tried to keep it light and humorous, and provide you guys and girls with links to follow-up on anyone thing that takes your fancy.

I'm currently writing a Fiction book based on an end of the world scenario and Sam is running her own company. I wanted a break from my novel and she wanted to work on something with me together. So here we are Being A Man is born. Consider this an idiot's guide to being a man. Tips, Tricks and Hacks and as much information on a variety of man related issues that we could fit into one book. You won't find out how to hunt a wild pig bare handed and then skin it with a rock but there is definitely something for everyone here.

So enjoy our hard work, read it sitting on the plane between business trips, on the toilet, or just when you have a spare 5 minutes. This book is intended as a light warmhearted attempt at passing on tips and tricks, with our opinions finely ingrained in them so please read it with that in mind. Please feel free to email us with any comments at benandsamauthors@gmail.com.

Thanks for taking the time to purchase this book and please enjoy it.

Ben & Sam

DATING MAN

THIS CHAPTER IS all about dating. There is so many different types of dating out there that depending on where you are in your life you might have come across some of these or none of them. So let's start with the easiest one of all.

Casual Dating: This type of dating has its good and bad points. It's for the people just looking for a fun time without any commitments, still searching for their soul mate or anyone looking for a good time. Depending on your reasons this may or may not work for you. But no matter what make sure you know what you are getting into with this, more hearts are broken because people aren't upfront about their intentions. If this is where you want to be for the time being, then make sure you are looking at the right type of woman. Don't try to casually date the woman who wants to settle down right away. Honesty is the best policy here, oh and make sure your being safe.

Speed dating: personally I never done it but there is plenty of this in bigger cities. Long and the short it's a common spot where people gather, such as bars and restaurants. Each couple has a set time to talk and see if there is anything of interest there, then you move onto your next partner. During the night people normally score each other and at the end people are matched accordingly. If you find someone interesting and they reciprocate contacts can be exchanged.

Blind dating: How many times have your friends told you I know the PERFECT person for you? Have you ever gone? Most people are terrified of these types of dates, with good reason. Depending on the person trying to set you up, I would seriously consider at least one date. What's the worst that can happen? Haha, okay in all seriousness there are some friends of mine that wouldn't know the first clue on what I like in a man. So make sure you let the right friends choose for you, if not I would probably not do it. But if you are in the right place and you like what you hear from your best friend then go for it, nothing ventured, nothing gained. Worst case you are back to where you started with a tale of the blind date from hell or you might have met someone you actually really mesh with. Quick tip on this always be wary of family members or particular parents trying to do this, unless you have a great relationship with them and I mean confident, best friend knows almost everything about you otherwise you will end up with a tale for the boys.

Double dating: This is pretty self-explanatory, it's great for couples just getting to know each other. But later on double dating and group dates are perfect for couples who already naturally hang out.

Serious (Committed) Dating: This is the BIG one, this involves just you and your girlfriend in a committed relationship. This is where some of the above leads to, which can end up in marriage.

A few hints from a woman's point of view:

1. Always be honest no matter what.
2. When you apologize make sure you know what you are apologizing for.
3. Tell her she's beautiful all the time. *(Please ignore Rule 1 if she's a hideous beast –Ben ;))*
4. Make each other laugh.

I could list hundreds but these are the important ones that you should always remember.

Online dating: There are many different forms of online dating. The most popular is dating sites, this is where people post a profile with a few things about themselves and a photo. (*Heads up if you want serious results be truthful if you don't look like Brad Pitt don't pretend you do - Sam*) (*Guys if you want any results, use a good camera angle - Ben*) After you connect with someone, photos, emails and texting/chatting are exchanged. Once you are ready you can then proceed to meet up. This is a great alternative for people who don't have time for conventional dating especially at the start of relationships.

Since we just went through the many types of dating I thought I would give you the top Do Not's of dating some apply to first dates more than others.

- Keep the conversations light don't go into anything serious, this applies to first dates and any newer relationships. No Go topics: Religion & Politics at least for the first few dates

- Ask questions don't be the person who just sits and nod at her

- Same thing make sure you are listening, and really listening. One of the most important parts is listening to what she has to say.

- Hygiene - !!!!! I can't stress this enough show up clean or don't bother coming at all. See my manscaping man chapter for a few tips.

- Always be on time – My suggestion here is to be at least 10-15 minutes early. I personally hate when people are late, but even worse when it's a date.

- Unless it's an emergency keep that cell phone away. Another self-explanatory thing. Follow my advice.

- Eye contact – if you are staring at her boobs instead of her eyes there's going to be a problem. But at the same time don't be creepy and stare too much.

- Confirmation before a date, don't just assume that everyone is on the same page. Send her a quick text or email or give her a quick call.

- Act like yourself - Don't show up acting like a show off this doesn't serve any purpose and she will think you're a tool, so be you and either she will like you or she won't but better than living a lie.

- Last but not least laugh, throughout any relationship there needs to be laughter if there isn't you will need to contemplate why you are truly there. Same note don't start off on the comedy circuit, just have fun and good luck

If you are anything like Ben he loves going out to do things but usually I do the planning, so when he does plan something I am so surprised and excited. These can be adapted to people who are a bit more serious to first dates, be creative.

Dinner & Movie - Great for conversation and some entertainment. If you're worried about conversation switch them around see the movie first so you have some conversation pieces for the dinner.

Picnic on the beach/secluded area of the park/or anywhere that sets a mood - The classic picnic date, may seem like its old and out of date. But believe me most woman would love to have their man show up with surprise plans and be greeted with this. Make sure your picnic basket contains all the important things – blanket, drinks alcoholic or non, depending on where you are, food: the key ingredient here is make it easy to eat sitting on a blanket but don't grab McDonald's make it yourself. Sandwiches, Rolls, Cheese & Biscuits or cold cuts.

Sports day – Not all woman will appreciate this date. But those sports playing woman will love it. Pick a sport you both love and plan the day around it. Here is a few suggestions, could be an afternoon baseball game followed by dinner, early morning drive with your surfboards to a beach, surf then have breakfast or brunch afterwards. To an evening hockey game with drinks afterwards. All depends on your special lady but I love sports days with Ben. Switch it up if you can, do sports dates with you as spectators and also sports days of you playing something sporty together even if it's mini golf.

Chef for a night date – This is the time to use some of the ideas mentioned in our Cooking man chapter. Invite your special lady over for a home cooked meal prepared by you and only you. Grab some wine or drinks, turn on some music and relax. *(Hint if you are a really horrible chef please don't try out the recipes for the first time on her, test it and conquer the recipe don't make her the guinea pig - Sam)*

Movie Night – This involves a few movies, blankets, couch, popcorn and some refreshments. These nights are easily the most popular and the cheapest. To make things more interesting play around with the movies. Don't always go for the new releases. Surprise her with some favorite old movies and some of yours too. *(Ben here, Sam and I did an outdoor movie night in Brisbane, got snacks, walked along the river, then chilled on bean bags in front of a big screen, was awesome.)*

Games Night – This night can take on a few different things depending on if it's a double date, group or just the two of you. Make sure you have some games around the house. There is a couple of websites with some of the top games for games night. But make any game into sexy time with your woman. Throw on some music and have a few drinks, relax and before you know it you'll be reminiscing and sharing stories from your youth. *(Ben and I are very competitive but makes for some great laughs.)*

Amusement park date – If you are lucky enough to both like amusement parks this is one of the greatest ways to spend the day. You both get to let off workweek steam and enjoy being a kid again while riding the rides and eating corn dogs and cotton candy. *(Ben here, I hate and I mean hate, roller coasters with a passion, but I still go on them with Sam every now and again. My eyes are shut and I'm white knuckled with fear but I'm there.)*

Once again I could go on and on but you get the general idea behind it. These are some of my personal favorites and depending on what you both like you can mix and match.

Dating can be scary and wonderful all at the same time. Believe me if you have read our bio then you know. So take some time, be prepared and have fun. Unless you want to grow old alone and live life on a small island like Tom Hanks in castaway, with only a soccer ball to talk to then get out there and mix it up.

Check out these websites for date friendly games:

10-board-games-couples-spend-time-together

best-adult-board-games/

RULES TO BEING WITH A WOMAN

I thought I would touch on this topic as some men have no clue how to talk to a woman. There is so many books out there to help you on this, but I am going to give you my views as a woman.

Pickup lines – For the love of all things holy please don't start off a conversation with some corny pickup line you saw in a movie or book. We can see those a mile away and the chances of you actually pulling it off are slim to none.

Be honest – If you plan on seeing this woman past the first date, start off by being honest. Don't tell her you have a Porsche then show up in your Honda on the second date, or tell her you're a lawyer and you flip burgers at McDonald's. Nothing wrong with any of those but lies will always catch up to you sooner rather than later

Future plans – This section I am adding because there are so many woman who get hurt months or years after being with a man because he forgot to mention some very big details. If you have no intentions of marrying or having children then state it upfront especially the older you get. At 33 years old if I was dating someone and after 6 months I have fallen in love, he blurted out that, I would be hurt and pissed. Doesn't need to be the first date but make sure you work it in if that's something you aren't willing to budge on.

Compliments – Always make sure that you compliment your woman. Always say she is beautiful, sexy, fine or however you want to say it but several times a day in person, on the phone or in a text. Make sure she knows that, woman love to know that their men find them sexy, whether you have been together one month or ten years.

I love you's – Same thing as compliments several times a day. Nothing beats an I love you from my man.

Family - When involved with anyone their family is now yours. All their little quirks and annoyances are now something you must learn to love. Tread carefully in how you talk to her about them. This is also a given with us to your family. Heads up if I am pissed and venting to you about my family, best suggestion is empathy. Never get in on the bashing I promise that will only turn out badly for everyone.

Kids – If she has kids, once again tread lightly here. Here is my suggestion as I have been in this situation personally. As noted in #3 if you aren't interested in her kids or having future children together don't go past the first date. If you are interested, then as things progress you will be introduced. Make sure that you know the mothers rules, don't be that boyfriend who is the class clown with them. This is very frustrating for the mother who then has to deal with the outcome. My best suggestion is take things slow, some will resent you and some will love you. Play with them, talk with them, listen to them and get to them as them. The first time that my children connected with Ben I knew without a doubt that he was the one.

DATING HACKS

- Have you ever wondered if that number she just gave you is real? Make sure before you leave you recite it back incorrectly. If she corrects you it's probably real, another way is to add it to your phone and call/text her right there. If she panics then it probably wasn't a real number.

- Most women want to hear how much you like them vs how they look. So make sure you compliment them on those things that they are skilled in vs how their hair looks. (Compliment her on everything but make sure she knows that you like her for who she is not just what she looks like.)

- If you are ever thinking of doing a cooking date night or even a second date make sure that you work it into the conversation so that you can surprise her with something special on another date.

- On the first date there is always an awkward pause at the end of the date about who's paying or if you are splitting the bill etc. So if you would like to avoid this before they bring the bill excuse yourself as if you're going to the washroom and pay the bill then.

- If you want to know more about your date then pay attention to how she treats the people around her. If she treats the service staff poorly or is rude to other people she doesn't consider as good as her then she will most likely treat everyone around her like this.

So we are going to cover a few different areas in this chapter. To start things off let's go to one of most popular.

FOOD MAN

MAN FOOD

OKAY HERE GOES, the most popular man food on the market! Well, some of them anyway I could go on and on and post a million different recipes here but I'm going to limit myself to some of the most popular recipes that would make any man's mouth water. I'm not posting all the recipes as all this book would be then is a cook book, but I will include some links, so that if any one dish gets your taste buds tingling you'll be able to get on the World Wide Web and find it for yourself. (just google each recipe by name)

Now, everyone has his own favorite recipe that he's made or someone else has made for him over the years and my personal absolute favorite meal is BBQ and Corn. I'll give you the recipe for the tastiest grilled corn you ever had and you can all thank me later. This Mexican corn recipe is easy to make and believe me, everyone will be asking you for the recipe. *(Sam here, what Ben actually means is you can thank me later) (Yeah, maybe, Sam learned the recipe in Las Vegas then changed it up, FYI I've been to Las Vegas since then and hers is better! -Ben.)*

PARMASAN ROASTED CORN ON THE COB

http://allrecipes.com/recipe/142410/parmesan-roasted-corn-on-the-cob/

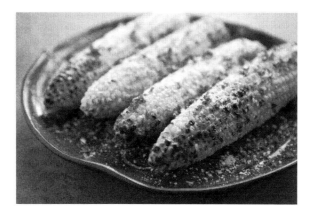

Next up on the list in no particular order is an all-time favorite, the classic Meat Loaf. Now everyone has tried it and sometimes it's not the greatest but this old time dish will get you back on the Meat Loaf train with this delicious recipe from The Pioneer Woman. *(Just a trick my dad taught me if you love cheese then do small cubes and add them into your meat mixture, makes a delicious addition to it – Sam)*

MY FAVOURITE MEATLOAF

http://thepioneerwoman.com/cooking/my-favorite-meatloaf/

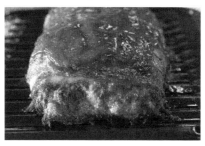

Moving along to our next delicious dinner time favorite we have Coca Cola ribs. Now I know what most of you are thinking, we all have our special way we like to cook ribs but just give this one a try and you won't be disappointed.

SWEET COLA RIBS RECIPE

(http://flavorite.net/2015/05/27/coca-cola-bbq-ribs/)

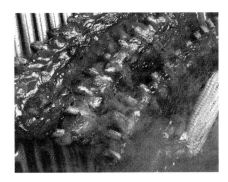

This recipe has a million different versions and is served all over the world made with every meat, or sometimes no meat at all, can you guess? If you guessed burger then you are 100% right. I'm going to give you a recipe for a hunger smashing Cheese burger here that will leave you satisfied and wondering why you haven't been doing this your whole life. This Cheese burger is from our old mate Jamie Oliver. *(This is one of those recipes that you can bring out for the guys as your own secret recipe at your next BBQ- Ben.*

ULTIMATE CHEESEBURGERS

http://www.jamieoliver.com/recipes/beef-recipes/
louie-and-gennaro-s-ultimate-cheeseburgers/

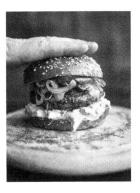

CHICKEN FRIED STEAK

http://www.myrecipes.com/recipe/chicken-fried-steak-3

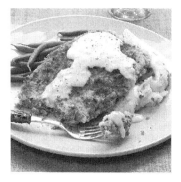

Now that I have your attention with some simply amazing meals we will move on to an absolute crowd pleaser the Chicken Fried Steak. You can serve this with veggies and mash or chips and a delicious rich gravy is an absolute must.

CLASSIC HOMEMADE LASAGNA RECIPE

http://www.simplyscratch.com/2012/11/classic-homemade-lasagna.html

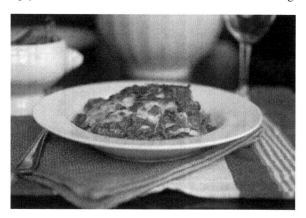

If you are looking for a go-to dish that you can pull out to impress or maybe just make ahead of time and keep in the freezer then you can stop looking right now. This classic Italian dish is definitely a favorite, you can serve it up with salad or vegetables, even just by itself. Yep, Lasagna, homemade delicious Lasagna. Believe me you'll never eat another store bought Lasagna after you try this classic recipe. *(Add in some homemade garlic bread and Caesar salad for a complete dinner-Sam.)*

BEER CAN BARBECUED CHICKEN

http://allrecipes.com/recipe/214618/beer-can-chicken/

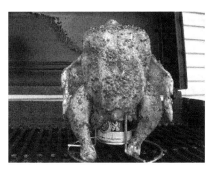

Nothing says man food more than the word "whole". This next recipe from myrecipes.com includes a whole chicken on the BBQ and will leave you wondering why you haven't been doing your chickens this way your whole life.

BEER BATTERED FISH

http://allrecipes.com/recipe/20107/beer-batter-fish-made-great/

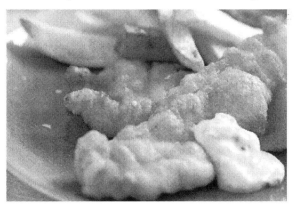

Now the best Man food recipes wouldn't be complete without a few popular recipes that have beer as an ingredient. The first one of those I'm going to give you all is one of my personal favorites, Beer Battered Fish and chips. You can't beat the flavor and freshness of catching your own fish and making a delicious meal out of it to feed friends and family. Here's a recipe that will get you started.

STEAK & GUINESS PIE

http://www.jamieoliver.com/recipes/beef-recipes/
steak-guinness-and-cheese-pie-with-a-puff-pastry-lid/

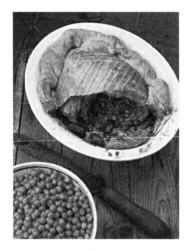

Next up our small trip along beer flavored treats is a Guinness Pie, now this recipe is courtesy of Jamie Oliver who has made it into the list once again. If you're English or Australian chances are you have had one of these and I personally have tried this recipe and it is just smashing. Sam, who is Canadian, had her first pie not so long ago and it was a Guinness Pie, and guess what? She loved it. Okay enough of me here's the link to the recipe.

What Man food recipe list would be complete without a Chili recipe. Here is a delicious beer inspired Chili recipe to warm you up on those cold winter nights.

CHILI RECIPE

http://www.pipandebby.com/pip-ebby/2014/2/15/the-best-chili-on-earth.html

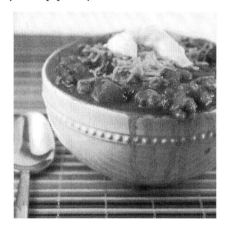

Okay I hope I have inspired some of you to dust off the apron and get into the kitchen and try cooking a meal for you or family and friends. Don't be scared to experiment either, if you find a recipe you like maybe try tweaking it a little to make it your own.

GAME DAY SNACK FOOD

So here goes with some super delicious recipe ideas that will hit the spot during your game day party or just any sort of social gathering where you're going to be drinking plenty of beer and need some good food to go along with it. I'm not going to post fifty different recipes here but just give you a brief description and any that take your fancy you can dig up the recipes. I'll try to break it down into smaller categories which will make it easier to plan what you want. When you're planning the party always remember to take into account how many people you expect and allow a little extra and make sure you have plenty of left overs for later in the day/ night for snacks or a late supper.

Let's start with some very simple **DIPS** and **SNACKS** now chili is always one of the more popular dips but just remember not every likes it hot so don't try to melt the enamel off people's teeth. Now you can't have a dip list without mentioning buffalo chicken dip, delicious nacho dip and a good old-fashioned favorite cheese dip. Here is a link to some delicious dips that are easy to make and all of them are crowd pleasers.

SUPER BOWL DIP RECIPE

http://www.food.com/ideas/super-bowl-dips-recipes-6236

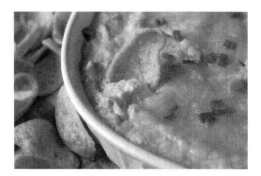

Now onto some bite sized **Finger Foods** for snacks that everyone can just eat one-handed so they can still hold there beer, sticky sweet or spicy wings, mini hot dogs, mini meat balls on sticks, party pies, sausage rolls, bacon wrapped smokies and last but not least classic mini pizzas. All of these can be made or bought before the party then just heat and serve during day or night as people want to eat them. Don't forget to keep the potato chip bowls filled up you can never ever have too much food around when there is football, beer and manly men around. *(A fun suggestion is a nacho bar, it's easy and fun. All you need is tortilla chips, nacho cheese, finely shredded lettuce, diced tomatoes, salsa, guacamole, sour cream and anything else you like on it. Put them in nice bowls and some plates and let the wolves at it – Sam)*

If you are looking for a more of meal then you can't go past **BURGERS/ SANDWICHES** to fill that hole in everyone stomach right to the top. Some great burgers are the classics, bacon cheese burgers, chicken burgers, ham and cheese melts, parmigiana burgers, egg and bacon burgers the list is endless and you can always make a few of each then let everyone pick their own meat and extras straight off the grill. Pulled pork and brisket sandwiches are definitely a crowd pleaser, they will cost you a little time in preparation but overall the praise is definitely worth that extra bit of hard work. Along with steak sandwiches and toasted ham and cheese melts, chicken and cheese or bacon all will hit the spot. A good sandwich for colder winter days is a roast beef or chicken, pork or turkey roll with gravy, just slow roasted and kept warm so they can be served up ready for whenever people want to help themselves.

If you are looking for something easier than you might want to go with **COLD SNACKS** as an option just make some sandwiches or wraps the day of and make sure to keep them refrigerated. Ham salad, bacon, cold burgers, Bologna, roast chicken let your imagination run wild, and just remember variety is the best option to cater to everyone's different tastes. You can also go with cheese and cold cuts platters, salami, kielbasa, cheeses, pickles and tomatoes. Veggie trays are always great too.

So there it is a variety of different ideas to help keep everyone's stomach filled, the more they eat the happier they will be and the whole day will be a huge success.

DATE NIGHT DINING

For those special dinners, there is plenty of meals I as a woman would love for my man to cook me. But it really just depends on what you both like. So make sure that you that you have some idea of what she doesn't like. Don't prepare a steak and potato if she's vegetarian, always make sure cook to what you know and to what you both will enjoy. No point cooking up a meal that you both won't enjoy. So I will give you a few different ideas that will make sure everyone is happy.

I won't make this into a cook book as I have told you before but I will list a few easy and tasty recipes that should be able to give you a starting place at least. Just mix and match things to what you both enjoy.

BEEF

Here is a few steak ideas that will hit most people's palates, check them out and remember what I said in the dating man chapter, don't try the recipe the first time on the date. Practice makes perfect.

SIZZLING SESAME BEEF

http://www.goodhousekeeping.com/food-recipes/a10191/
sizzling-sesame-beef-recipe/

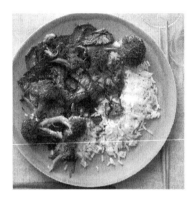

FLANK STEAK WITH RED WINE AND OVEN FRIES

http://www.goodhousekeeping.com/food-recipes/a7187/steak-oven-fries-2784/

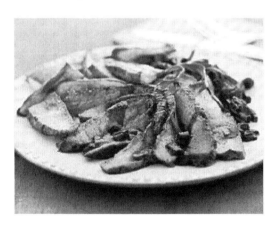

FILET MIGNON WITH ROQUEFORT

http://www.goodhousekeeping.com/food-recipes/a8936/
filet-mignon-roquefort-ghk0108/

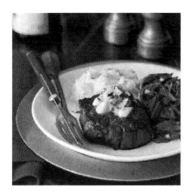

Here is a few protein packed meals some are harder than others so be mindful of your cooking skill level before you start.

OVEN FRIED CHICKEN WITH YOUR CHOICE OF VEGGIES AND STARCH

http://southernfood.about.com/od/ovenfriedchickenrecipes/r/r80320f.htm

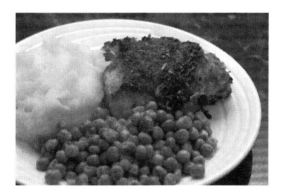

CHICKEN AND MUSHROOM WITH COUSCOUS

http://www.foodnetwork.com/recipes/food-network-kitchens/chicken-and-mushrooms-with-couscous-recipe.html

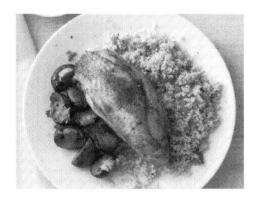

FISH

SEARED SCALLOPS WITH CREAMY MASH

http://www.jamieoliver.com/recipes/seafood-recipes/seared-scallops-creamy-mash/

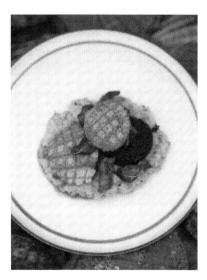

SPAGHETTI WITH PRAWNS & ROCKET

http://www.jamieoliver.com/recipes/pasta-recipes/
spaghetti-with-prawns-and-rocket-spaghetti-con-gamberetti-e-rucola/

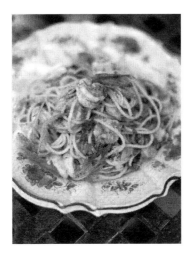

For those with a special diet here is a couple favorites

VEGETARIAN

GORGONZOLA PASTA WITH WALNUTS

http://www.tasteofhome.com/recipes/gorgonzola-pasta-with-walnuts

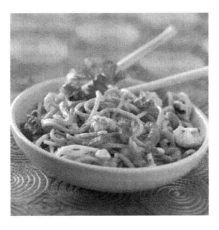

VEGAN

CREAMY AVOCADO 'CARBONARA

https://crunchandchew.wordpress.com/2011/04/06/creamy-avocado-carbonara/

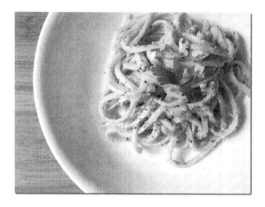

As for desserts let's be serious I could go on forever but seriously if you want to try to cook dessert on top of dinner all the power to you but I would be impressed if dinner was served not black, so for the dessert portion I would visit a local bakery and grab something small either in two portions or something to share.

FOOD HACKS

- Egg shells are an absolute pain in the ass, so if you are mixing her up some eggs for breakfast and you got some shell in there, little trick is to wet your finger with water. This makes the removal process that much easier. Or use the other half of the shell if it's not shattered and remove it with that.

- Check out ramsaysrecipes.com for how to cook a steak. Gordon Ramsay has been screaming his way across our screens for a few years now, take my advice read it he knows his stuff.

- Some people might not know this but if you add a wet cloth to the underside of your cutting board it can stop it from sliding around, this could save you some serious cuts to your fingers.

- Lemons & limes are very firm, to get the most juice possible out of each one roll them under the palm of your hand for a few seconds with a light but firm pressure. This will give you the most juice that can be used for cooking, baking or drinks.

- A neat trick to keeping your wine cool during those hot summer months is to freeze some grapes. If you are entertaining outside add 2-3 in each wine glass.

MAN'S MAN

GAMES NIGHT

SOMETIMES A MAN just doesn't feel like going out drinking and would much rather just hang out at home maybe invite over a few friends and play some good old fashioned drinking games. There are hundreds of different games from all around the world and I could fill a whole book just on those so I'm just going to list five of the most popular and there basic rules so that you can get together with your friends spill some beer and try them out for yourself. If any of them take your fancy there is several championship leagues out there with a detailed list of rules so that you can have a more professional game.

Probably the most well-known drinking games of them all is **BEER PONG** played using plastic cups half filled with beer and ping pong balls. Opposing teams take it in turns trying to bounce the balls into the plastic cups usually six or ten arranged in a triangle, two shots per person or until someone misses. Then the cups with balls are drunk by the opposing team and they then take a turn throwing. After each round teams are normally allowed to re-rack the remaining cups into a diamond or sword shape to make for easier shooting. There is several rewards throughout the game such as a bounced or deflected ball being worth two drinks and two balls landing in the same cup is worth three.

The next game in our list of international beer drinking fun is called **QUARTERS** and it's one of the easiest games to set-up and hardest to master. Players sit around a table and place a glass, full or empty your choice, approximately ten inches from each player. Then each player takes a turn trying to bounce a quarter off the table and into the cup, they make the shot they get to nominate someone to drink then they can shoot again, if they miss the next player takes a turn. You can add different twists in such as if you hit the rim you can re-shoot if you hit the glass three times you must chug..

Number Three on our list is **CASE RACE** a very simple game for when you just want to have a good old fashioned messy night. Teams of normally three race against each other to see who can finish their case first using any method that they like such as chugging, beer bongs or shotguns. The only down side to case race is that the better you are the shorter and messier your night generally ends up being.

Number four on our booze guzzling list of fun times is **I NEVER** and it's great for getting to know people or even among old friends just having a blast. Each player takes it in turn to start a true statement with the words I never for example, I never wet my bed when I drank too much, if any other players have done this they must chug their drink. Now there's no need for explaining just drink and move on! This game is best played honestly as possible it's a lot more fun and as the night goes on its just hilarious.

Last but not least lucky number five is **KINGZ** and all you need is friends a deck of cards and preferably a well-stocked bar! Start dealing out the cards one at a time to each player first one that gets a king picks the liquor next one dealt a king picks the mixer, third king buys the drink and lucky last gets to drink the either delicious or disgusting concoction! You'll need a strong stomach for this but just remember you could pick the gross drink or mixer then end up drinking it, Enjoy!

THE MAN CAVE

Now readers we are going to delve into a magical world, a hidden planet, that secret place where men all over the world seek refuge from the horrors and hardships of day-to-day life. That's right the man cave, that one place where a man can run away and hide and spend endless hours tinkering away or just laid back in a favorite recliner watching sport, a race or just playing a video game. There a many different guises a man cave can have and many different functions but the one essential thing they all have in common is the fact that they are a designated place where a man can go and get a break from life. Now don't get me wrong I'm not saying that we are over worked or our wives/girlfriends are so horrible and mean that we need a safe room just that It's nice to have a place where we can pursue our hobbies or just kick back and watch a movie or a game that no one else wants to watch anyway with the surround sound kicked up to register on the Richter scale. There are a lot of different manifestations of a man cave for example,

A Games Room = flashing lights and ancient PAC man is the first thing you notice then the pool table, pin ball machine, fooze ball, table tennis, dart board, air hockey etc.

Classic Man Cave = Think southern, antiques, cigar smoke, brandy and a few animals heads mounted over a roaring fire.

Motor Head Man Cave = You can smell gasoline when you walk into this secret garage, V8 coffee table, chairs made out of old car seats, NASCAR posters, engine parts, hot rod magazines and a bar made out of the front end of an old Chevrolet.

Tech Head Man Cave = Now we are getting into the realm of roof mounted projectors or maybe 80" flat screen TV's, a surround sound system that smashes windows and shakes foundations, iPod docks and a smattering of devices that look like something that NASA installed on the space shuttle.

Gamer's Man Cave = Similar to the Techies cave but with a whole lot more consoles, PS4, xBox1, classic Sega or maybe N64 with Golden Eye. All the things you wanted as a child and weren't allowed to have or couldn't afford.

That's a few different sorts of man caves and I could go into about a dozen more all slightly different from the rest but that's just a few of the more popular ones. Now every man has something that he collects or favors more than the other things in his cave maybe its coolers, vinyl records, number plates, hub caps, movie posters action figures and other endless lists of collectibles. Every man is different so what floats his boat might not necessarily be another man's cup of tea but when it all comes down to it, it's his man cave, his hideaway so what he puts into it is up to him.

MAN HACKS

Having a pool party, and don't want to play beer pong on the deck or lawn. Grab some peg board, pool noodles and string and put the noodles around it. Might need to use a few under depends on the weight and length of the board.

If you are having a night with the boys and your hanging by the fire worst thing is fishing through the cooler searching for a beer. Grab a few glow sticks and throw 1-2 inside to light it up.

Always carry cash! Sounds simple right, another thing that I need to do more of. Always have an emergency $20 note tucked away for those occasions when a card won't cut it.

The do's and do not's to a perfect handshake:

> **DO** - Maintain eye contact with the person that you are shaking hands with.
>
> **DO** - Lean forward slightly and shake from the elbow not the wrist, keep the fore arm rigid.
>
> **DO** - Make sure your hands aren't sweaty.
>
> **DO** - Five shakes MAX!
>
> **DON'T** - Crush the other person's hand. You are proving nothing.
>
> **DON'T** - Shake with just your fingers. Creepy Much.
>
> **DON'T** - Let you hand flop around like a dead fish. Gross.
>
> **DON'T** - Reach past the wrist with your fingers. It's just plain odd. Don't do it. Ever.

Every man will at some stage in their life need to kick down a door. Right? Damn right. If you haven't then you should, right now. Doors don't cost that much really, just smash one to know what it feels like. Before that though do it right, plant our back foot firmly, lean into the kick and kick right near the lock but not the lock itself. Make sure you are wearing adequate shoes for this or you may just break your foot.

MAN SCAPED MAN

FOR ALL INTENSIVE purposes we are going to go with my thoughts here, plenty of woman like different things but going with the majority. I will let Ben have a crack at it after but do remember MEN that a woman knows better especially in this department. Okay so where to start… *(Yeah I just do what she likes for the most part, although I have been growing a messy beard while I was away, much to Sam's disgust! - Ben)*

SHAVING

Okay so let's start from the head to the toes (yes I said toes). Some men have the knowledge in this department from girlfriends, sisters, books, internet etc… You men that haven't got a clue listen up. Shaving is one of the most critical things in the attraction department. For example, two different scenarios here. Let's use Ben as the man in question. He shows up on a first date looking all sexy in his jeans and shirt, (yes, there is some times this is appropriate). The woman in question thinks "man he looks hot". She looks him up and down. First thing she notices is his face in this scenario Ben has a short beard, it's nicely trimmed up. The date goes great. Let's fast forward as we don't want Ben sleeping with her the first date. The time comes for them to sleep together, as they undress each other she notices that he has hair on his chest. Not a huge deal as he doesn't look like an ape. Then she gets downstairs and notices that he is trimmed and shaved up. During that whole time she appreciates the time he takes to take care of himself. Okay so second scenario, Ben shows up in the same sexy jeans and shirt. But this time she looks at his face and notices that he has bushy eyebrows and a messy beard. In the back of her head ALARMS are going off. If this is what he goes out into public like WTF is hiding under those clothes. But his personality wins out. A little while later it's time to sleep together. She takes off his shirt and gasps because there is more hair on his chest and back than on his head. She recovers quickly but she's disgusted. He now takes off his own boxers and that's it she's done. He has never trimmed or shaved down there.

So I assume from that story you get it. But let's break this down from head to toes guys. Everyone will have certain ideas of what they like. Man scaping shouldn't scare you, so take it slow. These are the areas that you need to consider

> **Eyebrows** – should be neatly trimmed up. Using tweezers, eyebrow brushes you can do just that. If you can brush them they are TOO long. If you haven't done anything before to them I would suggest **http://bit.ly/1ECpFGi.** Worst case scenario you end up with one eyebrow. If you are man enough go spend the $10 and get them waxed, it lasts longer and they know what they are doing.

> **Nose & Ears** – short and sweet here disgusting if you can see it we can see it. So start looking at yourself in the mirror. There is plenty of trimmers that will take care of these, the older you get the more hair you will find heads up. Here's a good example of one **http://amzn.to/1hDEbmS**

> **Face** – There is so many different looks. The most important thing to remember here is make sure that it's always properly trimmed. If you wear a goatee or short beard, that's the key. You don't want to be the person with a crazy beard because that is exactly what you will look like walking around. Even people who wear long beards, all the power to them not my preference but make sure they are combed properly and you don't have random crap floating around it.

Chest – The most important thing here is trimmed up if you are one of those men that has long ass hair. You don't want to look like an ape so make sure you keep it contained. Plenty of men choose to shave their chest. This works but make sure you keep it up. Just like you hate prickly legs on your woman, we don't want to get a rash from your prickly chest. There is always the option of waxing or hair removal creams.

Down There – There comes a time when I am sure that getting hair there means you're a man. BUT… keep it contained guys. No woman wants to see more hair there then on your head. This means everything!!! Please don't make me paint the picture here. If the image of a golf ball with hair comes to mind then get it figured out ASAP. Most men can accomplish this with a beard shaver/ trimmer and a razor. .

Backside – No comment! Just a given. Would you want your woman to have a hairy ass? This is trickier as you can't see it, peach fuzz is fine. If you go beyond that call in a professional.

Legs – No need to shave your legs unless you are an athlete etc. But if you do just remember the upkeep in that. Woman hate shaving for a reason. If your legs resemble something out Planet of the Apes then might need to thin it out.

Toes - Last but not least. Most men wouldn't even think of their toes. A small patch is fine but it ends there so make sure you don't let it get out of control.

The Planet of the Apes reference works for a lot of men out there. If you are reading this and you have alarms going off as you read this. Then I suggest that you learn how to man scape for any future or current woman.

MAN SCAPING HACKS

- Do you always get razor burn? It sucks right. Try leaving your shaving cream on for 5 minutes before you shave.

- Any woman can tell you this neat trick, use your hair conditioner as shaving cream for those sensitive areas.

- Brush your teeth in the shower, saves time with no mess.

- Do you have a big date and a big red zit? Any Visine around the house? Dab a bit on to take down the redness.

- Use your nail clippers to trim moustache hair when you can't get to trimmers.

TECH MAN

IN THIS DAY and age it's all about the gadgets right? Hell yes it is! If you haven't got the latest phone, laptop, tablet, home entertainment system, games console, NAV man, motorcycle, car, boat or truck well you just aren't living right. With technology changing so fast it's almost impossible to stay ahead of the ever changing curve and unless you robbed a bank or own one then, let's face it, to most of us it's out of our reach. However, what we can do is try to stay up to date in most things or pick one and get the best one on the market no matter what it is. I'll try to give you a guide here on some of the best products on the market for 2014 and what's coming up in 2015. I can't write about everything so I will pick some out of our list and let you decide for yourself.

First on our list is something that you just can't do without, take calls, make calls, browse the World Wide Web and take photos, that's right **Mobile Phones.** Everyone has one, your granddad and grandma, even your kids have one these days and why wouldn't they. They are like putting your shoes on before you go out, you just pick up the mobile I personally would be lost without mine.

TOP 5 MOST POPULAR PHONES ON THE MARKET RIGHT NOW FOR 2014 ARE FROM 5 UP,

5. **iPhone 6 Plus:** Bigger screen, better camera and best of all a bigger batter but price puts it below its little brother.

4. **Samsung Galaxy Note 4:** Great display, awesome power supply and S-Pen lets you scribble to your heart's content but you'll pay for the pleasure.

3. **LG G3**: Excellent display and a removable battery and SD card are two great features an overall slick phone with an affordable price tag.

2. **iPhone 6:** Smaller than the plus but such a comfortable and sleek design. It does everything the others do combined but doesn't excel in any one area. Another great addition to the apple family.

1. **HTC One M8:** Great phone, comfortable and price wise the numbers don't lie. What more do I need to say.

Next things on our ever growing list of things that I would like to own but can't afford are one of my personal favorites, **Game Consoles**. Now there isn't a lot of choices and most people like to stick with a particular brand so for a first time gamer thinking of reliving your lost youth I'll give you a quick look at the most popular consoles and why they are at the top of the pile.

Sony PlayStation 4: There is a reason they have two games consoles in the top 5 they know what they are doing and the PS4 is no different. Best rating overall and has an easily up-gradable hard drive. The only thing really lacking is multimedia apps and video chat but I'm sure they won't be far away in the upcoming updates.

Microsoft Xbox One: The Xbox One has massive potential but falls slightly behind the PS4 in gaming.

Microsoft Xbox 360: Huge games range and massive entertainment apps on the 360, but the DVD player means a lot of new games need multiple discs to load.

Sony PlayStation 3: It has been replaced by its older brother but the huge range of games and free online play combined with its price still make the PS3 hard to beat. Blue Ray alone is well worth it. The only drawbacks are it's an old tech now so will be harder to source new release content for.

Nintendo Wii U: The tablet game play similar to the DS is good but overall it has hard to use online and lacks the simplicity of other consoles.

http://video-game-consoles-review.toptenreviews.com/

Okay the last product for Tech Man that I'm going to write about is **TV's.** I'm not going to try to compare all the different models, there's just too many out there on the market. What I'll try to do is give you a few different options and some of the best features of them all. There is a lot of choice now a days and your budget after all is going to be the deciding factor so only purchase what you can afford.

We will start with the size of the TV that you are looking at buying, bigger isn't always better and sometimes the size of the room directly effects the size of the TV you need. The size of the screen is measured diagonally from corner to corner and doesn't include the frame of the TV newer TV's have no edge or bezel or a very minimal one.

If you are looking for a TV to watch sports then you want to get a TV with a higher refresh rate this will ensure that you have less lag on those action games and movies. Extra HDMI ports are something else to take into consideration if you are running multiple devices such as Games Consoles, Blue Ray players and Surround Sound Systems.

3D TV's are all the rage and being able to sit back and watch crazy 3D movies in your own living room is something to think about if that's what you might be interested in. The latest thing to hit the TV market are Smart TV's so you can browse the web, watch Netflix or Cable and all just buy downloading an app. Your TV simply connects to the wireless network inside your home and then you can download apps and customize your TV to your own preferences.

4K is the best resolution on the market at the moment and as the name implies it's 4 x better picture quality than Full HD. LED TV's will give you a sharp, bright and vivid picture and are one of the most energy efficient models on the market. If you are looking for a larger screen you might want to look at a Plasma TV, great for action movies and sports they work best in larger darker rooms.

Well I hope that this gives you a better idea on some of the different Mobile Phones, Games Consoles and Televisions on the market and which one might best suit your needs.

http://www.argos.co.uk/static/ArgosPromo3/includeName/tv_buyingguide.htm

TECH MAN HACKS

- A great way to keep your cords organized with your bedside table or desk is to fit a power strip or board in to the drawers so that you can plug all your phone and tablet chargers in without having a thousand cords hanging over the place.

- Need some emergency speakers for that important game or race? Simple throw your smart phone into an empty red solo cup.

- If you are anything like me you're forever destroying the end of your phone charger cable. To stop it grab the spring out of a pen and place it over the end of the cable to stop it getting bent and twisted.

- If you let your phone battery run down to almost zero and don't have a lot of time left to charge before you have to go out, then try placing it on airplane mode to speed up the charging process.

- Before you send anymore weird blank emails, try working from the bottom up, write the message then subject and lastly put in the address. Presto, no more blank emails.

OUTDOOR MAN

OKAY THERE IS a lot to be said for getting outside and back to basics. These days us and our kids spend so much of our time inside either with work or just relaxing after work that it's easy to forget what we used to do growing up with friends and families. I remember as a young guy growing up that it wouldn't be unusual for me to go outside in the morning, grab my bike, and not come home until it was dark or dinner time. Now it's hard enough to get kids outside with the crazy amount of electronics that are available for them, and even find time for ourselves to get out and do stuff. I'm not the greatest camper or hiker but I do enjoy fishing and it's surprising how much exercise you can get in just a few hours fishing. I'm lucky though, I live close to the water and the forests and it's not too much of a stretch to be able to just pack a rod and hit the water. So let's try to break this down into a few different things here:

HIKING

We will start with hiking and branch off into the other two as we work through this I think. If you want to go hiking for an hour or a day there is a few things you will need to get you started on the right track (ha ha). Some people walk for a week others just prefer a short walk to see a certain feature such as a water fall or maybe a lookout. The first thing that anyone should do before setting off is planning, work out where you are going, how to get there and how long it will take. Now in this wonderful modern era that we live in all this information is just a fingers tip away from us. No longer do we have to rely on information passed on from a friend or an old map we bought at a gas station a few years ago. Get online, and find out exactly where you want to go, find out how hard the walk is, how long it will take and when you expect to start and when you'll be back again. Right, we know what walk we want to do, the where and when and the next thing we will do is check the weather forecast. Now, where I live, it can be raining one minute and sunny the next, then change again and we're back to pouring rain. So we get online, check the weather forecast maybe use a weather app on our smart phone or for old school people, watch the news the night before. Well now, we know what to expect from Mother Nature and all the details of where we are going the next thing to do is let someone know what we are planning. This is critical for your safety, tell them where you're going, when you should be back and make sure that they have your number and you have theirs. Even if it's only a thirty minute walk, always expect the unexpected and plan accordingly. This way if you break your ankle, at least someone will be wondering where you are eventually and be able to direct help to the appropriate location. Now for the love of all that's important to you, tell someone reliable. It's no use telling Steve if Steve's heading out on the town for a night on the drinks is it? Fat lot of good Steve would be. Moving on to the next part of planning, what to take for your walk. Here I will give you a quick summary of what you should take based on.

http://www.rei.com/learn/expert-advice/day-hiking-checklist.html.

Firstly you will need water, always take enough and allow extra in case it's warmer than expected or you end up being outside longer than you thought. Light plastic bottles are always a plus but these days you can get some great aluminum ones available at good outdoor stores or online.

Next up is food, take enough to keep you going and then a little extra, remember you have to carry whatever you bring so pack food that's high in nutritional value but low on weight. Granola bars, dried fruit and vegetables, nuts and even chocolate bars and energy bars.

Always take sunscreen, put some on when you leave and take enough so that you can re-apply on the walk. No matter if it's cloudy or not, being outside all day will leave you sun burnt.

Make sure that you have your phone if you get service, a map (I know right an old school piece of paper with directions on it!) and a compass if you can use it. If you can't then learn, here's a quick link and one day it might just save yours or someone else life. http://www.wikihow.com/Use-a-Compass

Wear adequate clothes! Take a light water proof jacket in case it rains, a hat, light long trousers or shorts and remember to be prepared for any weather.

A small first aid kit is essential for small walks or long. It doesn't have to contain much and you can either buy one or make your own.

Remember to take a small torch, these days you can get great little LED torches that take up absolutely no room and will get you out of trouble if you find yourself out later than expected.

Matches or a lighter is a must if you plan on lighting a fire or if you get stuck and its cold. No one wants to spend a night out in the cold but remember to always check the rules and regulations of wherever you're going to make sure that you can light fires.

Last but not least is a multi-tool, which should have a knife, pliers, tweezers etc. You never know what you will need it for but you will be thankful if it pulls you out of that hard spot you're in.

Okay that should get you out on the day trails and experiencing all that Mother Nature has to offer. There is a big wide world of pretty cool stuff out there and remember to take a camera with you and charge it the day before, believe me there is nothing worse than having to carry a camera around all day and not even being able to use it.

CAMPING

For camping we take can the basics we learned about hiking and expand on them here. More equipment to carry and more planning but longer to experience the outdoors. Plan your route! I can't stress it enough, work out where you're going, how long it will take, where you're staying and always allow a little extra time between stops. If you're a first time camper or not experienced try starting off nice and slow, pick a campsite with plenty of facilities available. If you have been a few times then try getting a little bit more adventurous with your trip, hike into where you want to stay or do a circuit trip staying at different places every night.

There's nothing better than spending a few days and nights in the great outdoors with friends and family. Just remember though you have to carry all your stuff in and at the end of the trip you'll be carrying it all out. How much gear you take will depend on how long and how comfortable you want to be. Some more serious campers take just the bare essentials but others like to live life outdoors with a bit more style. You don't have to spend a bundle on gear either but remember you get what you pay for and you are investing in equipment that has to stand up to a lot and last the distance.

Okay let's try and give you a quick list on what you will need to get you started on the first camping trip. I'm going to base this off beginners and assume you will be driving straight to the site and won't be hauling in all this stuff yourself. Just remember there is always a limit to what is really essential and after a point you are wasting money on stuff that might just sit in a dusty cupboard somewhere. A quick way is to go into an outdoors or sporting goods store have a look at what they're stocking then see if you can find the same brand online or elsewhere at a better price. Always remember if it's a new tent don't wait till you get to the campsite to try it out. Open it up in your yard and check because some need that extra coat of water sealant on the seams. This is the time to do it, I have had many over the years and even if they said it was fully protected I always do it again. And you also want to make sure you have everything and know how to set it up so you're not standing there looking like an idiot out in the forest.

First up the number one thing if you're camping overnight is a good quality tent. You have to do some research here as there is literally thousands available but take into account the weather conditions and how many people you need to sleep. Remember to take a ground sheet to set up the tent on, hammer and extra ropes and tent pegs.

Sleeping bags are pretty damn important unless you plan on sleeping in the cold! Same as tents do your research and buy sleeping bags that suit the climate and conditions. If you don't want to wake up with a crooked back then I suggest also a mattress of some sort. You can go with a thin but light foam roll up mattress or an air mattress. Just remember if you go with air to take a pump and patches, just in case you get a leak.

You can go two different ways when you are deciding on what you will be eating while you are camping, first take a cooking source or secondly precooked meals that can be eaten cold. I'm not going to go into all the different camping stoves but just buy one to suit what you will be cooking and remember to check on the rules of wherever you will be going.

Always pack enough clothes and assume the weather might change, that way you will be prepared no matter what.

Last but definitely not least, TOILET PAPER! Unless you fancy wiping with leaves and twigs then this one is probably the cheapest but can easily turn your trip into a nightmare if forgotten.

This site http://www.lovetheoutdoors.com/camping/checklists.htm has a great list of things you will need to take and all available in an easy checklist that you can print off to make sure you're ready.

When you have everything you need, you know where you're going and how to get there, and you told someone your itinerary you're ready to set up. First thing you're going to do, if you can some campsites have designated spaces, is choose where you want to setup. Pick a spot that offers you shelter from the elements and isn't right on top of someone else. Remember you'll be walking back and forth to shower and to the toilets so take that into consideration, you don't want a hike to the toilet at night.

Make sure the place you decide to setup the tent isn't too close to the fire and clean the area of all rocks and branches that could stick into your tent. Put down the ground sheet first and then setup your tent on top of it. The groundsheet will stop the bottom of your tent being ruined and also add protection from water and anything left on the ground. UN-pack your sleeping gear, mattresses and anything else like chairs and you're ready to go! Remember to be considerate of others camping and to keep the area clean and animals away always clean up and dispose of rubbish and food scraps in the areas provided. I hope you find this as enjoyable as I do and it will lead to many pleasant and sometimes hilarious stories to tell for years to come. This site has some great tips to get you started and remember safety first and always tell someone where you're going.

http://www.idiotsguides.com/sports-and-fitness/hiking-and-camping/camping-101-how-to-set-up-your-campsite/

OUTDOOR HACKS

If your camping and want to have light but only have a head lamp then consider this as an idea. Grab your head lamp and strap it to a gallon jug of water, it will give you a lot of ambient light without the harsh direct beam of the head lamp.

Make an emergency camp stove out of a soda can using only a knife!!! Okay I'm not explaining it as there is a video here Camp Stove Tutorial that does a much better job, but what an awesome idea and I'm going to make one myself right now!

Okay this might sound obvious but an easy way to make sure your gear stays dry in your pack is to just grab a garbage bag and use it as a liner. Simple and afterwards you can put your trash in there.

Another great idea is a product called a Life Straw. You can drink any water through it and it purifies it for you, a million people in Africa can be wrong. It retails for about $20 and lasts a single person a year on average.

An empty pill bottle makes the ideal holder for an emergency first aid kit. You can fit in antiseptic wipes, band aids, and headache pills. As an extra bonus wrap a couple of lengths of tape around the container to be used in an emergency, saves bringing the whole roll.

HANDY MAN

EVERY MAN ON the planet will at one time or another have to do one of several different things involving tools. Starting with your car there are many small things that you can do yourself to save paying expensive fees to tradesmen. Have you ever tried to get someone to come to your house to fix a leaking faucet at short notice? Then you have to pay through the nose for the pleasure. I will try to give you an easy guide to doing some of these things for yourself and a basic list of tools that will get you out of trouble.

CAR MAN

There are several different things that you can easily do for yourself to keep your car running and it will save you a few $$$ down the road. Many years ago in a time long forgotten we used to be able to pull up into a petrol station and have our oil and water checked, and the pressure in our tires checked and topped up. Those days of driveway service for the most part, are now long gone. There isn't any reason why we can't do it for ourselves though, and it's a good idea especially if you have a decent amount of time between scheduled services.

The best time to check your oil in the car is before you go for a drive while the engine is cold. This gives the oil a chance to level out in the bottom of the engine and will give you an accurate indication on the dipstick. Open the hood of your vehicle and find your dipstick, remove the dipstick and using a clean piece of rag or paper towel wipe the oil off the stick. Slide the dipstick back in and then remove it and make sure that the oil is between the minimum and maximum marks on the stick. If it's between these marks you're okay to go and won't need to add any oil, but if it's below the minimum mark then you will need to add some oil. Make sure you check the manual to see what oil you need to use then add a little bit at a time to make sure that you don't over fill it. If you put too much oil into your car it's bad for the engine and will also cause it to smoke a lot! You can buy oil from the gas station but it's normally cheaper to buy it at big outlets and keep it in your trunk or garage at home for whenever you need it.

Checking your tires is another easy way to save a few $$$. You wouldn't think so but driving around on tires that are flat is not only bad for the tires, but gives you low gas mileage as well. With the price of gas the way it is these days it doesn't take long for a few pennies extra too really add up. You can buy a cheap air pressure gauge online or from most hardware stores and keep it in your glove box, then every week or so just whip around while the car its warming up in the morning and you will be able to keep a close eye on whether the tires are low or not.

It's recommended by most tire businesses that you rotate your tires at least every time you get your oil changed, if not more often. With the right equipment, such as a Car Jack and Jack Stands, you can easily do this for yourself and once you have done it a few times it won't take you long at all. Rotating the front and rear tires prevents over wear on the front which means you'll get longer out of a set of tires, and that means you will save some money! Win on that right. Please make sure that you use decent certified Jacks and Jack Stands and you have a level place to jack your up on.

How often have you driven past some poor guy or girl that's parked on the side of road with a flat tire just scratching their head and waiting for help to come? Too often. I never wanted to be that person and hopefully after reading this you won't be either. With the right tools changing a flat is pretty easy, make sure your spare is always pumped up and you have a Jack and wheel wrench. Most cars, especially new ones, come with all the tools you need, but if you buy a used car then double-check everything is there. Here I'll give you a quick point by point guide to changing your flat tire.

If you're driving and get a flat tire then find a safe flat spot as soon as possible to pull over in. Also make sure that whatever road you are on allows this. If you're just driving through you can take a chance but major highways are usually a no change zone. If it's at night time then try to find somewhere well-lit like a car park.

Always when you're stopping like this place your hazard lights on to warn other motorists that you have stopped.

Get all the tools out you will need, jack, wrench and spare tire. Make sure your spare is pumped up.

Start by loosening all the nuts on the wheel, but don't loosen them completely off.

Now place the jack under the edge of the chassis of your car or if it's a jack specifically for your model of car there will be a locating hole to place the jack in. Jack up the car just enough so that the wheel is able to freely spin around, remember the flat is skinnier so allow for that.

Remove the nuts off the wheel and place the flat tire off to one side, grab your new tire and line it up with the studs and slide it on. Put the wheel nuts back on and tighten them all finger tight.

Once you have all the nuts done up finger tight then lower the car down and start tightening the nuts but don't just do one all the way, spread it out so that you make sure the tire is on equally.

You're all set to go, make sure that you put all the tools back away and drop the tire off asap to get it fixed and back on the car.

Okay now you're changing tires like a NASCAR pro, just be aware most new cars have spare tires that are a specially designed spare, that isn't designed for long distances or high speeds. It always pays to practice anything so why not have a go changing your spare at home where it's nice and comfortable.

HOUSE HANDY MAN

It's always handy to have a set of tools for around the house or apartment. You don't need to be a qualified trade's person to be able to do a few basic home improvements. It doesn't need to break the bank either, these days there a lot of cheap tools that will get most jobs done and still be there for the next emergency repair. If you are considering bigger projects then invest in quality tools, life time guarantees are just that, if it breaks they'll replace it for you. Your basic tool kit should include the following:

The first thing on the list is a **Claw Hammer,** get a decent weighted model without going crazy, and remember you have to be swinging the bloody thing. You can use this hammer for hammering in nails, and then removing them, and for smashing just about anything.

A **Screw Driver Set** with a Flat Head, Phillips Head and a Robinson aka the square head, in a variety of sizes will cover you for 99% of most jobs involving screwing anything. Some screws use a different pattern and you may have to buy specific tools for that screw, but they aren't very common in day-to-day jobs.

An **Allen Key Set** with both imperial and metric keys is the way to go, don't go crazy, just buy a set that has half a dozen of each and you will be fine.

Adjustable Wrench is next on the need to have list. The name implies it all, a wrench that you can adjust to suit a wide variety of nuts and bolts. There is also a bit pricier version that I have that includes a ratchet for sockets and a hammer edge for when subtlety has gone out the window.

Socket Set is something that will definitely be handy. Don't go crazy and spend a fortune but a decent set is something that you will still be using 50 years from now.

A **Cordless Drill** and **Drill Bit Set** is something that everyone should have one of. These days with the new lithium-ion batteries they charge super quick and last a decent amount of time.

Tape Measure. Well you can't measure anything without a Tape Measure. Cheap and bright colors so you don't lose them every 5 minutes. My suggestion is don't go for the super cheap ones they end up breaking.

Utility Knife or **Blade** is another handy quick tool but please keep them closed and keep them away from the little ones fingers. You don't want to be sitting in an emergency room explaining to your wife or girlfriend how little Sally cut her fingers off.

Some **Pliers** are a really good idea. I recommend a set that includes your standard pliers, needle nose and a lockable set of pliers.

A **Level** is pretty important bit of kit if you're building anything substantial, you don't want the leaning Tower of Pisa in your back yard, and you don't want to listen to hours of your partner trying to explain why something doesn't look quite right.

Lastly is a decent **Hand Saw** or **Power Saw**. Just be careful with either because fingers don't grow back no matter how much you wished they would.

Look after your tools and they will in turn look after you when you need them. Keep them somewhere safe and dry, store them in their boxes or in a decent tool box or bag. Leave them where you know where to find them in an emergency, they won't be any good when the toilet is flooding or a door is blown off if you can't find them.

Okay so we have mastered our cars and trucks, and now we have a pretty decent tool kit to fall back on around the house. Look after all your gear, keep it away from the kids! Not just for safety but because remember when you were a kid and ruined your dad's tools? Well now they're yours and you know what it costs to replace them! Don't be afraid to ask a friend if you know they are a bit gifted with the tools, get them around, help them out and learn for next time.

HANDY MAN HACKS

- Ever hit your finger or thumb while hammering in a nail? Of course you bloody have. Grab a clothes peg and hold onto the nail with that. Saves you some serious injuries to your digits.

- Got a stubborn screw that's been stripped to death? Try using a rubber band to get it off.

- Ever wonder why your lights are so dull when driving at night? You might not need new bulbs maybe you just need to clean of up your headlights. Use some toothpaste and it will polish and remove that haze off the glass that is making them dull.

- Another foam noodle trick is if you have a narrow garage and you or someone else you live with are always banging the car doors on the wall. Try cutting a pool noodle lengthwise and screw them into the wall where you normally hit your door. Works well on poles in carports too.

- Do you have a few dents in your car? If they are small in nature then grab that plunger from next to the toilet and put it over the dent and plunge away. It will pop it straight out, only works on small dents but it's better than nothing.

FITNESS MAN

CAN'T DO A man's book without a section on fitness can we now. Everyone has their own workouts and routines for staying in shape or getting in shape so I will just try and throw a few brief routines and tips and tricks in here. If you're anything like me and maybe need to lose a few pounds and are always struggling with weight then hopefully this helps you out.

First off we will try to focus on certain areas and some easy ways and cheap ways to stay in shape without melting the credit card completely. Remember the proper equipment is a must, just like any sport or activity if you aren't setup properly from the start then you won't get the most out of it. The really important thing is shoes, spend the money and buy yourself a good set of athletic shoes. Do some research and find what you will be focusing on and get the shoes to suit the activity. This is one thing I would recommend getting a professional to do, get decent shoes and have them fitted by an expert.

GYM MAN

The first and probably easiest way to keep in shape is by hitting the gym, the problem is always getting the time to go out and do it and some gyms are really damn expensive. This is going to be a newbie guide to gyms so if you're already smashing the gym sessions this probably won't benefit you much. Find a gym that's convenient for you, if it's close to home, or on the way to and from work then you will be more likely to actually use it. Find one with a pricing plan to suit your budget, most gyms offer free trials so take advantage of that and try out a few first see what you like. If you sign up for a year at some place you despise then you are destined to fail.

I'll start off with what you need to bring, not a lot just a few necessary items.

A must have is a water/drink bottle, remember you'll be sweating up a storm if you're doing it right and it's a must to replace those lost fluids.

Which brings me to the next item, a towel, if you're like me you will probably be pretty damn wet and remember other people have to use that equipment just like you do. (Most gyms supply towels it depends on whether or not they do so check that out)

Last one is some music, most gyms these days have plenty of music or televisions pumping out the tunes but personally I prefer to listen to my own tunes.

Okay, so we know what to bring to the gym what's next? There is heaps of different work out machines available in gyms so if you don't know what it's for ask an employee! That's what they are there for after all. Most gyms have personal trainers available and many offer beginner courses or even as part of the membership plans. Don't be afraid to ask, everyone was a newbie once upon a time and a little bit of courtesy can save you a lot of hassles or injuries down the track. If you want any more tips to gym etiquette then **http://bit.ly/1VztJeR** That should get you in the door and on your way to becoming a regular gym junkie.

HERE IS A SOME BASIC THINGS TO GET YOU STARTED

Now for some quick ideas you can do at home with the basic gear that won't break the bank. I will add in a few different websites with great workouts for home at the end of the chapter. If there is some things you can't do or don't like swap them out with another exercise that is that muscle group.

Weights are a good way to build muscle and a decent set won't cost you an arm and a leg. Dumbbells, weight benches, kettle-bells and you can even take advantage of what you have at home and make your own. Make sure if you are buying new weights get what you can lift, don't get 25lb weights if you can't lift more than 1. Lift a few up and try to get a range of what you can handle.

A skipping rope is a great way to get some quality cardio in and will cost you very little. It's a great cheap investment for the amount of work you will get done. Grab your phone and put your timer on, or use a song and skip till it's done. Great way to burn calories.

Exercise balls or medicine balls are cheap and easy. Exercise balls are great for many things, you can add them into any weight training exercise. They make your body balance which in turn makes your muscles tighten as you do it. So in saying this it's great for abs. Medicine balls are easy to use, but are expensive to have too many. Grab a ball that you can get 12-15 reps out of. Try doing medicine ball slams, or replace a dumbbell with it for an exercise.

Stair climbs just using the stairs you have at home will cost you nothing. Find some stairs with 10-15 of them, set your timer on your phone, start off with what you feel is comfortable for you. Sprint up the stairs and catch your breath on the way back down, jog or walk at a quick pace without falling. Be careful, continue at this pace. You can do this as a part of your cardio, you can do intervals with stair sprints and jumping jacks or push-ups whatever works. It will burn calories and having you sweating that fat off. (I *made Ben do this when we were living in Brisbane together, he hated it but was competitive enough to want to try to beat me - Sam*)

Walking or jogging will only set you back the cost of decent running shoes and it's something that you can do as much as you like. Also a great way to get some time in outside. Make sure you start off slow, go and grab a walk to run 5k app for your phone. This will give you a good schedule on how to get to 5k with less chance of injuring yourself.

Last one is just common sense really, grab a workout DVD (there is millions to choose from) and from the comfort of your own home you can do some serious workout sessions at times convenient to you. (Sam here, I have tried a ton of workout DVD's so rating them top 2 in my books, with some links.)

Shaun T's Insanity was my first real DVD workout unless we count Richard Simmons when I was younger. This workout almost killed me the first day but the intervals is what burns the most calories. Most won't be able to keep to their pace that's fine work at your own and move forward. This wouldn't be a suggestion for anyone just starting out, it's hard core but make it your goal. www.beachbody.com (He also has a few other DVD's that I have heard great reviews on some shorter and some sports focused. But all super intense)

Rip 60 is the next on my list, this is a variation of TRX system, which is just as unique of a workout but I found I liked the Rip 60 better. One of the biggest draws for me with this suspension trainer was that it was so easy to use. There is a few different variations but one of things I found was the TRX is stationary unlike the Rip 60 which you can take the pin out and do rotational work. http://www.proform.com

 Here is a link with some more videos for different things.

http://www.livestrong.com/article/120265-workout-dvds-men/

http://ca.askmen.com/top_10/sports/top-7-workout-dvds-for-men.html

No matter what you are planning on doing, make sure you check in with your doctor if you have any health issues.

http://www.muscleandfitness.com/workouts/workout-routines/
complete-mf-beginners-training-guide-0

http://www.mensfitness.com/training/workout-routines

FITNESS HACKS

- Protein is a must for anyone working out. Most trainers will tell you in general to always try to eat as close to one gram per pound of your body weight.

- Try Tabata, if you are running low on time. You can download an app. This involves a 4 minute workout-routine with 20 seconds work hard, 10 second break and with a complete 8 rounds all up.

- Log the food you eat, use an app like MyFitnesspal to keep yourself accountable for what you're eating. This will let you know where all those extra pounds are coming from.

- Eat with a smaller plate, sounds stupid but you will eat a normal portion size by doing this. It will keep you from overeating.

- Slow down when you eat at meal times. Let your brain tell your body when it's full. This normally takes 10 minutes so just give it a chance.

PARTY MAN

AS A WOMAN I know the horrors of an unorganized party. I have been to plenty of them where it's not even at the half time show and food dishes are empty, and the drinks are running low. You don't want to be that host, because no one will forget it. So here is some do's and don'ts at making your next game day party a success.

Make 2 lists – One for things to do and one for to buy list.

Don't Offer If your place is crap - Don't offer up your place for the biggest sports day of the year if you have a television made in the 1980's. Make sure it's big enough for your audience and that everything is working on it. 50 inches plus works for most parties.

Seating areas – Not everyone sits the whole time, but don't invite 25 people over to watch the game and only have couches that seat 3. Make sure you have plenty of comfortable couches and chairs with enough room for at least 75% of those people coming. Large pillows can be tossed on the floor too as an option.

Food – Won't say much here except have plenty of it, more is most definitely better, and always make sure your guest can get to it easily. See Cooking Man Chapter for recipes that will make sure everyone goes home happy and stuffed.

Drinks – Okay depending on who the audience is and how well you know them, be sure that you provide a range of beers and spirits. No need to go specialty beer unless you are keen too, just make sure you have the most popular beer brands and grab at least 1 light brand. Make sure there is vodka coolers or even some wine for the non-beer drinkers. Last but not least make sure you have enough for the whole time! Always make sure there is plenty of water and pops around for people who don't drink.

Glasses or plastic cups - Depending on the ages of the parties, I am going to suggest actual glassware for it. Nice pint glasses, highball or similar for mixed and wine glasses. This brings the class back into some parties if you are having a bit more casual then go for the red solo cups. But beware, that it looks like a college party vs an adult party when these are around. Your choice.

Pick your Guests - Your guest may include a wide range of people, but make sure you are comfortable getting really into a game in front of them. During games emotions tend to run high for most fans, you don't want to lose your temper in front of bosses or kids for example.

Decorations - Decorating can happen or not depends on what kind of party you want to have. But if you are supporting the _____ then throw some colors around. Or show support for each. Spice things up make the party exactly that.

Cleaning supplies – Make sure that you have plenty of paper towels and all-purpose cleaner around for those spills. If you have carpet in that area, make sure you have a rug cleaner on hand for those salsa spills. Remove rugs if you can, it will make your life easier at clean up time.

Get People Involved - If there is a football pool going on but not everyone invited is in it. Do a mini game grab a white board, chalk board or Bristol board and write down everyone's guess on the final score. Have a small gift for the winner! Example a Case of beer.

Have Fun - Last but not least have fun game day parties can be a blast be creative. I am posting some websites that have some great ideas to make your party the one everyone will talking about.

PARTY HACKS

- Did you know that those lines on the Red Solo cups actually mean something? The first line up from the bottom is to show you where a shot of spirits is, the second line up is for wine and the next line up is beer.

- If you're crowded for space when your cooking did you know that you can throw your corn on the cob in a cooler and pour boiling water over it!

- A quick and easy way to keep your drinks cool is to make water balloons and then freeze them, just throw them in a cooler with some water. Looks great and they will last longer than ice cubes too.

- You ever spend half the night at a party looking for a bloody bottle opener? Yep of course you have. Just tie the bottle opener to a piece of string and attach it to the handle on the cooler. Problem solved.

- Ran out of cooler space? Easy fill up the washing machine with ice and you have an instant cooler. Just make sure you unplug it!

CONCLUSION

SO THERE WE have it. There is a millions things that we could have poured onto these pages, especially me (Sam). One of the biggest issues as I got older was so many men that look like they haven't watched a show, read a book or listened to a female friend. I feel like walking up to some guys and giving them a slap to the back of the heads. I have been with a few men that for some reason or not think once they land the woman that they can just get lazy. Heads up it doesn't work for us on you so why would it work for us? You don't have to be Channing Tatum in the looks department. Think about that ridiculous show Beauty and the Geek that could be you hidden under that scraggly hair and beard. And the same clothes you wore in high school or college. No matter what your goal is in life single man or married man, you need to be armed with the basics. This is what we tried to provide from both the male and female perspective. If it's listed in this book with any regards to woman it means I support this fully. Not everyone will be MacGyver but with a little help you might be able to impress some friends, family or that special someone in your life. We hope you enjoyed it and watch for our Woman Hacks book coming soon.

RESOURCES

Many websites we used are listed at the bottom of our chapters the rest comes from years of experiences in this crazy world of ours.

http://thechive.com/2014/09/08/18-manly-life-hacks-every-guy-should-know-18-photos/

http://www.buzzfeed.com/readcommentbackwards/40-creative-food-hacks-that-will-change-the-way-yo-dmjk#.mfBBlZGDk

http://mancavedetails.com

http://www.buzzfeed.com/peggy/things-you-must-have-in-your-man-cave#.tpO2QbraZ

Some useful websites for decorating, games, food etc.

http://www.pinterest.com/pcrichardandson/game-day-decorationparty-ideas/

http://jennysteffens.blogspot.ca/2011/09/game-day-tailgate-party-recipes-decor.html

http://www.campbellskitchen.com/entertaining/big%20game%20day/5%20game%20day%20party%20tips

OTHER BOOKS BY SAM LAWRENCE & BEN JACKSON

Long Distance Relationships

Divorce Recovery

Prepper Items for SHTF Survival

The Before

Printed in Great Britain
by Amazon